Also by Dr. Stenbeck

Available from the usual on-line source

Books

Healing Yourself -- The Holistic Approach
   [An introduction to Holistic Self-healing.]

Heal Yourself Right Now!
   [The Seven Priority Organ Levels for
      effective Nutritional/Holistic Treatment of
      all organs.]

The 22 Unique Body Types
   (for Health and Weight Loss)
Q & A to Identify your Body Type (Booklet)
(Individual Body Type Booklets are available)

Booklets
(Step-by-step instructions on healing yourself)

   #1 Start Healing with Positive Thinking
   #2 Mastering Positive Feelings for Health!
   #3 Spiritual Balance and Your Healing

———

The Pathoferic Body Type

The Gwyneth Paltrow, Blythe Danner Celebrity Body Type

For Kaye,
there at the beginning with Doc Severn,
and for Liberty,
continuing the holistic healing journey…

Disclaimer

The information in this book is for educational purposes only and is not a substitute for medication, diets, or other medical care. The diets do not treat diseases or medical conditions, and are an adjunct to your orthodox health care.

The author and publisher accept no responsibility for any misuse of the information within. If you have any physical problem, food allergy, emotional disorder, or disease, common sense dictates that you consult with a physician before changing your diet, taking nutritional supplements, or following the advice given here.

———

About the Author

Educated in New Zealand and in the U.S.A., Dr. Stenbeck attained B.Sc. (NZ), M.S., and D.C. degrees. His holistic healing methods have been profiled in magazines (Esquire, McLean's, Playgirl, the Atlanta Constitution), and on TV in the USA and in Canada. He was the main contributor to the Warner Book, _The Eye/Body Connection_ by Jessica Maxwell that focused on the holistic healing relationships between the iris structure and organ genetics.

In the 1970-80's he was elected Fellow, Royal Society of Health, London; Fellow, American Association of Chemists; Member, American Association of Clinical Chemists; and Affiliate, Royal Society of Medicine, London. He studied naturopathy and Body Types with Dr. Bernard Jensen and Dr. Clifford Severn, and has practiced in medical partnerships where patients received the joint benefits of medical and holistic healing.

He is a member of Self-Realization Fellowship. To receive advice on any health issue from a holistic viewpoint, or to receive help with your body type, see his web site: *DrStenbeck.net*

———

Information follows the type description on:

> *Types, Minerals*
> *Researchers Genetics, Types, Diet*
> *Help identifying your body type, or with an online health consult with Dr. Stenbeck*

———

Contents

* * *

The Pathoferic Body Type (and Food Guide)   1

---

* * *

The 22 Body Types:
Celebrity Examples

This Booklet contains the **Pathoferic** *type.*
[See The 22 Unique Body Types *for all type descriptions.]*

Thin Types

Atrophic *Woody Allen / Audrey Hepburn*
  Stan Laurel / Calista Flockheart

Exesthesic *Cher / Sarah Jessica Parker*
  (Female type only)

Marasmic *President Obama / Princess Diana*
  James Stewart / Kate Blanchard

Neurogenic *J.K. Simmons / Joan Rivers*
  Jon Cryer / Marin Hinle

Pathoferic *(No celebrity males)*
  Blythe Danner / Gwyneth Paltrow

Sillevitic *David Bowie / Shirley MacLaine*
  Rod Stewart / Carol Channing

Muscle Types

Calciferic	*Michael Jordan / Angelica Huston*
Carbogenic	*George Clooney / Lady Gaga* *Pres. G. Bush, Jr. / Meg Ryan*
Desmogenic	*Marlon Brando / Loni Anderson* *Daniel Craig / Tina Turner*
Eldic	*Ross Perot / Hillary Clinton* *Peter Falk / Sigourney Weaver*
Myogenic	*Pres. Bill Clinton / Sharon Stone* *Pres. John Kennedy / Julia Roberts*
Nervimotive	*Frank Sinatra / Elizabeth Taylor*
Nitropheric	*Ben Affleck / Ava Gardner* *Kirk Douglas / Kate Winslet*
Pallinomic	*Pres. Donald Trump /* *Attorney General Janet Reno* *Bill O'Reilly (Fox) / Jane Russell*

Fat Types

Barotic   *Robin Williams / 'Mrs.Doubtfire'*
                Elton John / William Conrad

Carboferic   *Bill Murray / Roseanne*
                Billy Gardell / Melissa McCarthy

Hydripheric   *John Goodman / Shelly Winters*
                Wayne Knight / Jennifer Holliday

Isogenic   *Einstein / Oprah Winfrey*
                Phillip S .Hoffman / Queen Victoria

Lipopheric   *Rush Limbaugh / Rosie O'Donnell*
                Chris Christie / Camryn Manheim

Oxypheric   *Winston Churchill / Orsen Welles*
                Ella Fitzgerald / Gerry Spence

Pargenic   *Burt Reynolds / Katey Segal*
                Ron Perlman / Kirstey Alley

<u>*Succinct Quote on Human Types*</u>

From Victor Rocine, who first described discrete body types around 1900.

"A type is an order of people that differentiates and distinguishes itself by a general and similar form, brain-formation, chemistry, structure, build, immunity, tendencies, predisposition, resemblance, skin-pigment, and type characteristics based on observation and analogy.

"Or, in other words, people of a given type are similar physically and like-minded as if they were brothers and sisters—that is what type means.

"Everything in nature is made according to plan. Man only discovers that plan and gives it a name. The zoologist has not made the animals—he has only described the plan adopted by the wonderful Creator, and named the classes, subclasses, etc.

"How important type research will be to humanity, time alone will make known."

———

Prologue

The esteemed scientist J. J. Berzelius, discoverer of several chemical elements, inspired Victor Rocine to research body types and to investigate the correlation between types and their diseases. Around 1890-1910, Rocine privately published his original findings on the mineral basis of different body types, and this present book exists because of his brilliant insights.

For many years, I studied with Dr. Clifford Severn who had been a personal student of Victor Rocine on body types, naturopathy, herbology, iris analysis, diet, and nutritional healing methods. He had a successful career as a lecturer and healer, and was one of those rare athletes with complete muscle control over his body. I saw him under a spotlight at 85 years of age, contracting and rippling every individual muscle in his perfectly developed body. Field-Marshal Jan Smuts, the WWII South African Prime Minister, devoted a full chapter of his autobiography to how Severn's healing methods had saved his life. In the 1950's, *Life* magazine did a four-page spread on Severn and his family. Fame he had.

Another Rocine student I studied with, Dr. Bernard Jensen wrote of Rocine's body type research and nutritional methods in his privately published book *The Chemistry of Man*.

This book is deeply rooted in Rocine's original work, and with that of Herbert Shelton, M.D., Ph.D. (at Harvard University in the 1930's). I integrated their research with newer dietary and nervous system data along with celebrity examples of each type, hopefully, making this material easier to digest and more entertaining for the reader.

Gayelord Hauser, another Rocine student I knew, was a celebrated health book author. He wrote a popular book on Rocine's types in the 1940's, *Types and Temperaments;* reputedly, he also introduced yogurt to the western world.

This book exists because of Rocine's creative brilliance and original discoveries in natural healing.

▶ *Rocine: "The soul creates the body type."*

Rocine taught that the soul chooses a body type and brain to live in, thus presenting different experiences and life lessons to master. Why were *you* born the way you are?

That is something to think about, especially if it is true! What would your soul purpose be to live in a particular body type. I provide some thoughts on this issue in each type description and try to assess from my experience with your type the particular lessons of life presented therein.

Rocine was as brilliant in his way as an Abraham Lincoln, Michael Jordan, Michael Phelps, Tony Robbins, or a Daniel Day Lewis—all *calciferics*—rare, leaders, innovative, brilliant, and highly intelligent in their different fields of endeavor.

Celebrity examples exist for most types, not a duplicate of you, but someone who has your essence in their body-mind individuality. Knowing your type allows you to become a better you!

The celebrity examples provide further help in identifying your body type.

▶ *Rocine's classic findings are the backbone of this book. Integrated with Sheldon's research and with other dietary and food issues including mental, emotional, and spiritual attributes,*

Many people take nutritional supplements and try different diets without a doctor's advice. If this is your choice, use common sense, listen to body responses, and discontinue any allergic reactions to foods or nutritional substances.

———

The Pathoferic Body Type

Representing one of the 22 Body Types first described by Victor Rocine around 1900

* * *

"You may also have a physical or psychological feature not representative of your type such as height, weight, appearance, talent, weakness, strength, etc., due to biochemical errors, environmental influences, racial or cultural differences, and congenital or genetic issues. Nevertheless, the type identification of the average persons is usually clear."

— Victor Rocine

Celebrity Examples

If you think this is your type, be sure to look at **on-line photographs** *of these examples. Look for general similarities to yourself. Note that sub-types cause the differences in appearance between members of the same type. The scarcity of examples speaks to the rarity of this type.*

———

ACTING   *[There are no male celebrity examples.]*

Gwyneth Paltrow
Blythe Danner (Gwyneth's mother)
Claire Bloom (British)
Dana Wynter (British)
Kasha Kropinski (Ruth in Netflix: "Hell on Wheels")

The males have insufficient ego, drive, and aggressiveness to become celebrities; I know one man who became an assistant symphony director. The females, however, have their talent, beauty, intelligence, and a sweet disposition to propel them in successful careers.

[Note: I personally knew one of the above celebrities, and others in everyday life, which contributed to my understanding of the type.]

SPORTS

This type has no star athletes, as there is little muscle power or endurance. To do ten pull-ups, push-ups, or to run a hundred yards is a major achievement! I have known you to be average tennis players.

HISTORICAL (from Rocine)

Lillian Gish (Silent movie star)
Elizabeth Barrett Browning

You already know something about this type from their public persona and appearance, whether from seeing them yourself or from the celebrity examples. Blend such insights with the type descriptions and the types of your family and friends to discern their presence midst! Read the types, and if still confused, consider using the request for type identification from my web site: *DrStenbeck.net*

———

Pathoferic Type Questionnaire

These questions describe the generic type, and not specifically you! If any question ever applied to you, then choose the True answer!

For question 1 only:

A = True	*B = Maybe*	*C = Untrue*
15 points	*7 points*	*1 point*

1. Physically identify with celebrity example

         ____

Then...

A = True	*B = Maybe*	*C = Untrue*
5 points	*3 points*	*1 point*

---

2. Height is close to:
   Males: 5'8-5'11   Females: 5'4-5'8   ____
3. Weight is close to:
   Males: 140-170   Females: 110-140 lbs ____
4. Slender, proportional, attractive body   ____
5. Muscles weak; little standing strength;
   cannot lift own body weight   ____
6. Forehead retreating (particularly males) ____
7. Pleasant face, no cheekbone
   markings; chin smaller   ____
8. Teen acne may occur into adulthood   ____

9. Sensitive, small, and weak teeth, some discolored (need cosmetic dentistry)   _____

10. Not addicted to cigarettes, alcohol or drugs (have high self-discipline)   _____

11. Emotionally and spiritually sensitive   _____

12. Easily hurt; difficult to share emotional pain   _____

13. Tend to place other people's feelings ahead of own (co-dependent)   _____

14. Need a serene and happy home environment   _____

15. In marriage or love give without expectations   _____

16. May have low self-esteem and self-confidence   _____

17. Have a strong spiritual basis to life; aware of the God within; attracted to meditation and metaphysics   _____

18. Should avoid hard physical work (are a mental type)   _____

19. Lack leadership and management ability   _____

20. Goals and dreams outweigh ability to manifest them   _____

21. Are unselfish   _____

22. Are congenial and sympathetic   _____

23. Respect other people's viewpoints   _____

24. Disgusted by aggression, coarseness, shouting, unkindness, and violence   _____

25. If angered become sad, withdrawn, and walk away   _____

26. Well-mannered, polite, gracious, and
     peaceful   ____
27. Appear calm, but are often nervous   ____
28. Passive, rarely assertive, non-aggressive____
29. Refined, polite, generous   ____
30. Romantic and demonstrative   ____
31. Modest (low self-image)   ____
32. Rocine: "You are angelic…"   ____
33. If accused, decline to defend self   ____
34. History of fingernail white spots
     (zinc deficiency)   ____
35. Low will-power   ____
36. Conservative with alcohol and drugs   ____
37. Skin weakness: acne, moles, dark
     spots on skin are common   ____
38. May experience loss of taste, smell   ____
39. Have few gestures; controlled,
     restrained physical expression   ____
40. Rarely argue or raise the voice; walk
     from arguments; forgive too easily   ____
41. Appear youthful, shapely, harmonious   ____
42. Head is longer from front to back
     (especially males); large forehead with
     humanitarian lines (males)   ____
43. Hair is mostly light or dark brown,
     soft, fine, and luxuriant   ____
44. Need privacy, solitude   ____
45. Eyes weak, sensitive, often blue or
     hazel with arched eyebrows   ____
46. Nose may be larger than average   ____
47. Softly padded face   ____
48. Highly self-conscious   ____

49. Soft, sensitive skin (acne common in childhood) _____

50. Voice is sweet, tender, sympathetic, friendly, soft (never loud, rarely shout) _____

51. Smile, but rarely laugh _____

52. Show great secretiveness of feelings; suffer emotionally in silence _____

53. Very sensitive to noise; need peace and quiet _____

54. Feel unimportant (many wall-flowers) _____

55. Humble, shy, slow to converse, some socially impaired _____

56. Are loyal and devoted; usually have few close friends, but may have a number of acquaintances _____

57. Shy, high embarrassment level; difficult to communicate on an impromptu basis _____

58. Have tolerance, devotion, loyalty, and patience _____

59. Tactful, diplomatic, peace-makers; see good in people, refuse to criticize or judge others; have no enemies _____

60. Feel intellectually inadequate, lack general knowledge, may have special-ized knowledge; don't promote self _____

Scoring

For question #1:
A response: give 15 points = _____
B response: give 7 points = _____
C response: give 1 points = _____

For questions #2—60:
A response: give 5 points = _____
B response: give 3 points = _____
C response: give 1 point   = _____
Total of the above points   = _____

Interpretation
155—285: **PROBABLY Pathoferic type**
81—154: POSSIBLY Pathoferic type
<81: NOT Pathoferic type

The Pathoferic Type

Rocine: "Pathoferic means 'full of pity and sentiments.' Your weak <u>zinc and calcium</u> metabolism makes you sentimental, affectionate, warm-hearted, and romantic."

––––––

Y ou have weak zinc and calcium metabolism, are slender (or medium-sized) and of average height or moderately tall; you appear youthful, and have weak skin and teeth. You are devoted, gentle, loving, creative, mental, studious, sensitive, and sentimental; you may be sedentary and withdrawn, co-dependent, self-conscious, and excessively forgiving. You have an opposite mind and behaviors to the "macho" males found in several muscle types.

► *Rocine: "You are delicate in nerves and muscles. You have a romantic nature. You are genial, true, hopeful, faithful, friendly, graceful, beautiful, amiable, polite, cultured, agreeable..."*

You are often sickly when young; you know no malice, dislike raising the voice, have low assertiveness, and may be excessively accepting of other people's negative behaviors.

▶ *You are most unhappy if causing pain or being forced to argue with someone: you will walk from an argument rather than be involved in what you would consider denigrating, destructive, or unspiritual activity.*

Pathoferic minds are sedentary and designed for mental pursuits; you are spiritual, loving, and creative. You are rare, and feel different to the average person. You are congenial, introspective, often emotionally overly-sensitive and caring of other peoples' feelings. You crave peace and quiet, and enjoy work in serving others. You are soft-muscled with moderate physical strength: you do not like cleaning carpets, moving house or laying concrete! Hard physical work leads to unhappiness and exhaustion. You willingly do the dishes and pay others to do the gardening! Rocine originally called your sentimental type, *pathetic,* pejorative in the political correctness of today, which demanded a softer title, *pathoferic.*

▶ Rocine: *"You have no mind, body, or soul for battle—you are a peace-maker. You forgive, forgive, and forgive again."*

———

Physical Similarity to Other Types

The *marasmic* males may have similar features (like Leslie Howard and Richard Chamberlain).

► *Your type is rare in the USA, being more commonly seen in Scandinavian and British countries. In Southern California, I see mostly females of your type, perhaps only one male to 20 females.*

———

Average Height and Weight

Males:	5'8-5'11	140-170	pounds
Females:	5'4-5'8	110-140	pounds

———

Pathoferic Type Description

The type description represents how you appear in everyday society. You may have a sub-type that alters parts of this description.

Head — Your head is medium-sized, higher in the back-head with a prominent retreating forehead.

Hair — You have fair or brown hair with a fine, soft texture.

Eyes — Mostly you have blue or brown eyes.

Ears — Your ears are of average size and shape.

Nose — The nose is often larger than average.

Neck — The neck is thin and not strong.

Mouth, Lips and Voice — Your mouth and lips are normal-sized and balanced. Your voice is soft, controlled, and friendly.

Face — You have a softly padded face; the jaw-bones are not readily evident; the chin is normal-sized or smaller, without the indentation seen in most muscles types. The beard, if present, is usually shapely. Females tend to be sweet and lovely; the males attractive, quiet, and withdrawn.

Teeth — Commonly you have weak teeth and gums; cosmetic dentistry is helpful (also in the *atrophic, sillevitic* types).

▶ *You may have small unhealthy teeth due to sluggish calcium and/or fluoride metabolism in childhood.*

Skin — Soft, sensitive and youthful skin is usual. An incorrect childhood diet may lead to skin diseases or imperfections that last throughout life. After suffering with childhood acne, your complexion may be clear or always be a problem. Zinc and calcium are keys to your healing (along with releasing emotions like self-hate and self-disgust from the skin).

Muscles — Your muscles are small and weak; aerobics, light exercises, yoga, and isometrics are helpful, but your muscles respond little to weight-lifting. Your thighs and low back are usually strong. You are 10-20 times weaker than muscle types and cannot lift your own weight overhead. Light exercising, dancing, tennis, etc., are more your forte.

Chest — A small to moderate bust; the males show light chest hair growth.

Shoulders — You usually have rounded shoulders.

Abdomen and Hips — The abdomen and hips may become heavier with age and a poor diet.

Arms and Legs — Your extremities are lean, and of average length or longer; the upper arms are fleshier in the females; while the arms are weaker, your thighs and legs are stronger.

Joints —Small joints of moderate strength are typical.

———

Pathoferic Personality Traits

If you are this type many, but not all, of the following characteristics are present—you may have overcome or moderated the negatives, but recognize that you once had several of them.

Positive Qualities

- Are tenacious
- Are a strong mental type
- Need privacy and solitude
- Are honest and law abiding
- Are devoted, loyal, tolerant
- Are cultured, tactful, tender
- Sentimentality is a strong qualities
- Readily believe people are honest and good
- Strong in patience, modesty, respect for others
- Embrace change if it is not emotionally threatening

- Are non-combative, non-aggressive, and will rarely fight
- You are silent when hurt; may need assertiveness training
- Gestures are absent; physical expression is controlled and restrained
- Moderately high sex drive; capable of celibacy if true love not available

▶ *Rocine: "You forgive any injustice and are reluctant to defend yourself when wrongly accused: God's judgments are your only concern."*

- Respond to inner guidance rather than external influences
- Prefer indoor activities and mental pursuits: reading, TV, writing, arts and crafts, computer, etc.
- Have a strong spiritual basis to life and awareness of God; embrace meditation and metaphysics
- Are tactful peace-makers; see the good in everybody and refuse to criticize others; unlikely to have enemies
- Are humble, reticent, slow to engage in conversation; in friendships you are loyal, devoted, and usually have only a few close intimate friends

- May feel intellectually inadequate in general knowledge; may be brilliant in your chosen field, but do not like to talk about it (or to blow your own horn)

▶ *Due to high self-consciousness, you smile but rarely laugh out-loud.*

———

Potential Challenges

▶ *Rocine: "You are not equal to hardships, strife, fighting, quarrels, and argumentation. You need someone to do the hammering and to take charge of mean responsibilities."*

You may have evolved from or have not experienced these potential challenges, so do not dwell on this list:

- Are self-conscious
- Have postural awareness
- Prefer to suffer in silence
- Have limited management ability
- May feel unimportant around peers
- May be sentimental, fearful, cautious
- Have low assertiveness, willpower, ambition

- May suffer with shyness, and feel awkward in social situations
- You may not answer, or will walk away if someone is impolite, loud or inappropriate; it is very difficult for you to speak loudly or to scream

▶ *If you relate to any of these challenges, doing something to overcome them serves your evolution.*

———

Pathoferic Stress Management

You have moderate mental stress prevention providing a good ability not to internalize this stress into your stomach, adrenals, and immune system. Emotional stress prevention is not strong and any of the above challenges may need reprogramming help. Rocine said you are "full of feelings" and that is your challenge: not to allow emotions to overwhelm your rational mind. *[If needing help managing these stresses see Booklets #1 and 2, andor my prior books.]*

———

Love

You rarely fall in love, perhaps a few times over a lifetime. You are very sentimental. You are usually attracted to the *nervimotive, carbogenic, nitropheric, and myogenic* types.

▶ *In relationship disagreements you do not fight: you walk away feeling crushed, embarrassed, and humiliated for having upset someone whom you love or care for. You never deliberately upset or hurt anyone.*

You have low priorities on having many friendships; you have a small group of close friends and in this sense, you are born to be a reclusive or monastic, and probably are found in monasteries and religious retreats throughout the world.

———

Talents and Vocations

Abilities – *Scientific, artistic*

You are academically competent and tenacious, and through hard work often reach your goals. You do well in science, drugless healing, teaching, computers, education, the arts, and service occupations. The type information cannot predict what or who you will become, but you are capable of bringing a creative excellence or brilliance to whatever you do in life.

▶ *You want to help people—not sell, hurt, confront, convince, or persuade anyone to a particular course of action: you believe in free will for all.*

Inabilities – *Orthodox medicine, law, physical labor*

You are never a laborer, trade worker, or sales person. You have difficulty selling yourself, let alone your work product. You cannot be a dentist, physician or surgeon, and do not aspire to any work requiring strength of body. You are not lawyers or found in high executive positions, places of power, or any work requiring confrontation, or any job where others may be hurt by your actions.

▶ *I have known or observed you as waiters, healers, and in the teaching, and scientific industries.*

———

Health Problems

You may have allergies like corn, nuts, shell-fish, cruciferous vegetables, and black pepper; you are often lactose intolerant. Retained negative emotions may underlay the allergies.

► *Remove allergic foods from your diet, or suffer with hand, wrist and joint pains, fatigue and moodiness, acne and skin rashes, disturbed sleep patterns, and other disorders.*

If sick, you commonly experience health problems or diseases in any of the following organs:

Sexual Organs — Fibroids, cysts, and prostate problems are common.

Eyes — Are weak, easily stressed, and sensitive to light.

Skin — Your skin is usually weak, with acne and skin disorders common (often precipitated by self-negative feelings).

Adrenal, Liver, Pancreas — May suffer from hypoglycemia with fatigue, moodiness and headaches (due to negative emotions and diet).

Bones and Joints — Bones, joints, teeth, and gums are genetically weak and require nutritional attention; you may have difficulty utilizing bone nutrients (osteoporosis is common).

Chronic Infections — Sinuses, throat, and bladder are weak and vulnerable to infections (particularly in females).

———

Pathoferic Acid/Alkaline Factor

For your health and healing, the genetics of your autonomic nervous system predispose you to needing a specific ratio of food acidity to alkalinity. You are born with an alkaline constitution, which means you need a predominantly **acid-ash** food intake for acid/alkaline balance. (Ash refers to the minerals left in your body after metabolizing foods.) Your autonomic nervous system genetics are *parasympathetic* dominant, requiring about 70% proteins and carbohydrates, but...

For your healing, if in ill health or after about age 45-50, you need to aim for this approximate ratio of food selections:

50% Fruits, salads, vegetables
50% Proteins, carbohydrates

▶ *Approximate your food ratios. On any particular day, it does not matter if one meal is mostly alkaline and another mostly acid—just try to balance it out for the day! If you make a mistake, try again tomorrow. It is a subjective call that you make, and what is done over time that makes the difference to your health.*

────

The Pathoferic Spiritual Factors

Skip this paragraph if uninterested in a philosophical perspective on your body type!

▶ *Rocine: "The soul chooses the body type."*

If as souls, we choose the brain and body type to spend a lifetime in, it could be to learn certain spiritual lessons related to perfecting ourselves, and our humanity, in God's eyes. What lessons does the type bring you? Only you can really decide what those lessons are. You know your weaknesses, faults, and behaviors towards others. You know things about yourself that Victor Rocine could never get from his research subjects when he first wrote about types. So search your mind for the answers. Each discrete type has challenges of life lessons, spiritual goals, etc., and some of yours may be:

Oneness with God — Expand your developing faith and trust, and embrace an enhanced intimacy with God.

Social — In engaging others, realize that we are all equal in God's eyes.

Assertiveness — Develop an assertive nature instead of living in your inherited passivity around people.

Self-Negative feelings — You usually take on many childhood self-negative feelings like low self-esteem, image, worth, value, confidence, etc. Overcoming such feelings is vital to your happiness.

Mental Strength — Perhaps, most importantly, develop and nurture your mental body, your conscious mind, so that your life decisions are determined by right thinking.

High Self-consciousness — Acting, public speaking, and emotional maturity helps you evolve through your weaknesses.

Non-engagement — You may be as solitary as a monk in the cloisters or in the wilderness:

practice engagement with others! In fact, you may wish you lived in a monastery.

Low Assertiveness — You are passive, rarely assertive, and never aggressive; you need assertiveness training: karate and acting help tremendously!

Weak Willpower — Low will and ambition makes it difficult for you to make your mark in the world.

———

A Pathoferic Story...

Lenny, age 28, had suffered with acne on his face, neck, chest, and back since he was 13 years old. This was still humiliating and embarrassing to him and he was fatigued, moody, and frequently depressed. Examination revealed a lean body. His diet was appropriately high in carbohydrates and proteins, but too high in beef with a gross absence of high zinc foods like herrings, whole wheat, and oatmeal.

He also released negative emotions of self-hate and disgust from childhood pain with his parents, made the necessary corrections took supplemental zinc and made immediate progress. His skin, and his good feelings about himself soon shone forth. Attention to his *Food Guide* maintained his healing.

———

Pathoferic Type
Mineral Food Needs

Apply this mineral data to the diet following the Thin type descriptions

Excessive Foods:

- *Nitrogen (beef)*
- *Carbon (simple sugars)*

Deficient Foods:

- *Zinc, Phosphorus, Iron*
- *Calcium, Potassium, Iodine*
- *Nitrogen (non-beef, vegetable)*

These deficient nutrients are common deficiencies in your type, and predispose you to ill-health. If ill, be sure to use these lists with your daily food intake. If not ill, eat from the food lists 3-4 days weekly for health maintenance. All food lists are in descending order of concentration and value to you; choose servings of foods in the upper half of each list first! One serving is ½ cup.

Pathoferic Excessive Foods –

Nitrogen from red meat (if eaten more than once or twice monthly) is excessive in your diet and contributes to your acidity and illnesses. Genetically, you are a moderate carnivore, invariably craving or desiring flesh proteins in your diet: have eggs, fish, poultry, 3-5 times weekly.

Carbon, found in every cell of the body, is the basis of all life; you may eat it excessively. Avoid simple sugars, corn syrup, and fructose.

———

Deficient Foods -

In illness or disease, it is important to correct these probable mineral deficiencies.

Zinc is invariably deficient in your type requiring you take such foods and supplements (along with vitamin B-6 and hydrochloric acid).

Phosphorus may be deficient in your tissues, because of intense thinking and worries, and brain exhaustion.

Iron may be deficient in your tissues, especially in females. It is essential for absorbing oxygen through the lungs, and is active in many metabolic chemical reactions. Iron deficiency causes anemia with fatigue, and pallor.

Iodine may be a common deficit, causing underactive thyroid function.

Calcium is invariably deficient in your type. It is highly concentrated in bones, joints, muscles, nerves, heart, teeth, and gums. If ill or diseased in any of these tissues, calcium deficiency is a significant healing factor.

Potassium is often deficient in your type. It is concentrated in and vital to the health of your muscles, heart, brain and all cells. If ill or diseased, potassium may be essential for your healing.

Nitrogen (see above note)

———

<u>Minimize</u> Excessive Food

Nitrogen (beef):

Beef and red meats: 1-2 times/ <u>month</u>

Carbon: 1-2 servings/week

All simple carbohydrates, white sugar foods, high fructose corn syrup, white breads, sweet fruits, fats

Note -

The food recommendations are for the generic type. Additionally, you may need from a holistic healer or nutritionist something more specific for your individuality.

Eat
Deficient Foods

Zinc, Phosphorus, Iron:
1-2 servings/day
Herrings, sardines, brewer's yeast, seeds, rye, whole wheat and oats, millet, parsley, pinto beans, dried prunes, raisins, artichokes, lima beans, buckwheat, barley, lentils, peas.

Calcium, Potassium, Iodide:
1-2 servings/day
Kelp, dulse, blackstrap molasses, rice bran, Swiss and cheddar cheese, turnip greens, almonds, brewer's yeast, parsley, flour tortillas, dandelion greens, sunflower seeds, raisins, watercress, dried figs, sesame seeds, rice polishing, dried prunes.

Nitrogen (non-beef):
Eggs, poultry, fish —3-5 times weekly

Note: Eat any foods you desire, but be sure to include the type foods in your daily choices.

Pathoferic Nutritional supplements

- **Multi-Minerals —**
  [Take all supplements with food.]
  2 capsules/day (containing iron and zinc)

- **Calcium —**
  About 1,200 mg/day (not carbonate)

- **Omega-3 —**
  2 soft gels/day

- **Kelp —**
  4-6 tablets daily, two weeks; then
  2-3/week

- **Herbs —**
  Brain detox — Chickweed or Gotu Kola
  Organ detox — Red Raspberry or Strawberry
  Leaf
  (Take one capsule, twice daily for one month;
  then one, three times weekly.)

- **Lecithin —**
  About 1,300 mg/three times weekly

Important Pathoferic Health Concerns

Animal proteins should be limited. Usually you have milk lactose intolerance, and need to take 'lactase' with all dairy foods: milks, butter, cheese, cream, ice cream, etc. Excellent calcium sources for you are vegetable and fruit juices. Your nervous system genetics do **not** require the *vegetarian* Food Guide.

▶ *You require the Muscle type diet (Chapter 23) with more acid-ash foods than alkaline-ash foods daily.*

Any instinctive carnivorous cravings are normal and healthy as long as you do not overdo it! After about age 45 you need less flesh with about four flesh days and three vegetarian days each week. You need flesh, potassium foods, green salads, and vegetables in your diet. You are *not* born to be a vegetarian, but if you choose to be one be sure to take a supplemental protein drink (20-30 grams) each day.

<u>**Pathoferic Food Guide**</u>

Aim for:
50% Proteins, carbohydrates
50% Fruits, salads, vegetables
and
30% Raw food diet
70% Cooked foods
Take the recommended supplements.

▶ *You may be allergic to: GMO foods, MSG, corn, nuts, black pepper, and dairy foods (take with 'Lactase').*

Pathoferic Weight Loss

Losing weight depends upon you following the type instructions, summarized in this section, which is addressed by reducing calorie intake.

- *Eat* your body type mineral foods daily
- *Follow* your *Pathoferic Guide (as above)*
- *Exercise*: your body type requires moderate daily exercise (sports activities are best)

- *Simple sugars*: stop all white table sugar and high-fructose corn syrup and drinks containing these sugars
- *Calories:* As with any dietary approach, calories in, must be *less than* calories out! Most markets sell a calorie booklet; make notes of your daily intake, and in most instances keep it under about 1500 calc

———

Pathoferic
General Food Guide

(Carnivore)

Important Note

The Food Guide addresses the <u>Acid-Alkaline</u> aspect of your food intake, along with the <u>Type Mineral</u> factor presented throughout this book. It does <u>not</u> necessarily address calories or other dietary factors that may be pertinent to your personal health needs whether medical or appropriate for some other dietary need. So use your common sense and just include the factors described here with whatever healthy dietary choices you usually make.

For other nutrient information, consult with nutritional books or with holistic nutritional doctors. In this regard, I particularly recommend the advice of Andrew Weil, M.D.

Pathoferic
General Food Guide

This chapter presents a general Food Guide, upon which you superimpose the nutritional information from your type chapter. You are a Muscle type, your genetics requiring protein foods everyday. [Some of you, females particularly, choose vegetarianism.]

———

Meat/Flesh Intake

You should limit red meat to once or less weekly, while eggs, lamb, fish, or poultry are excellent in moderation. If ill or diseased, be sure to eat daily, one or two servings from each *deficient minerals* list. If not ill, eat them at least three times weekly for health maintenance. If this diet is similar to your present diet, but healing is sluggish, then:

- Decrease your carbohydrate and protein intake by about one-third
- Increase your fruit, salad, and vegetable intake by about one-third
- Consult with a holistic doctor, preferably one versed in nutritional and emotional evaluation

———

Over-Acid or Over-Alkaline?

Just as a log of wood burned in your fireplace leaves a mineral-ash, food ash refers to the minerals remaining after metabolizing foods in your tissues:

- Fruits, vegetables **alkalinize** tissues
- Proteins, carbohydrates **acidify** tissues

Usually You Are Over-Acid Due To:

- Excessive intake of dairy foods
- Excessive intake of proteins and carbohydrates
- Deficient intake of fruits, salads and vegetables
- Accumulated metabolic waste-acids (from years of eating excessive acid-ash foods, meats and carbohydrates, and from lack of exercise)
- You need to estimate the ratio of foods eaten. Generally, eat the following *approximate* ratios for your health:

50% **Alkaline-ash** foods *(fruits, salads, vegetables)*

50% **Acid-ash** foods *(complex carbo-hydrates like starches, grains, cereals, breads, flour products; and proteins)*

Approximate your food ratios. On any particular day, it does not matter if one meal is mostly alkaline, and another mostly acid—just try to balance it out for the day! If you get it wrong, try again tomorrow. It is a subjective call that you make, and it is what you do over weeks, months, or years that make the difference—not on any one or two days.

Note - If Vegetarian

As a general indication, if you follow a vegetarian diet substitute vegetable sources of protein for the any flesh in the food guide. Note that contrary to most alkaline-ash vegetarian diets you need something different:

*You need an **acid-ash** vegetarian diet high in complex carbohydrates and vegetable proteins.*

Because of your high need for protein, you usually require a vegetable powdered protein supplement in juice (about 25-35 grams daily).

Important

- Minimize white sugar and alcohol intake.
- If desired, interchange lunches for dinners.

- Never eat foods you are allergic to, no matter what I recommend; if allergic, or suspect a food allergy, eliminate it and substitute from your type mineral lists.
- Eat the right foods 80-90% of the time and the Food Guide will work for you; unlike some types you do not have to live out of a health food store (although such foods are healthier for you).

▶ *Omit eating the excessive minerals in your type chapter, and be sure to eat one or two servings from the deficient list daily.*

Finally, in addition to your body type needs, other holistic healing matters also need your attention. I strongly suggest that you refer to my web site and earlier books for that information: *DrStenbeck.net*

———

Acid/Alkaline Genetics Chart

The following chart reflects each Muscle Type and its acid or alkaline-ash food needs. These ratios change if you are unhealthy or over age 45-50. Refer back to your body type and review the *Acid/alkaline* instructions.

———

Acid/Alkaline Genetics, Dietary-Ash, and Raw Food Needs

This chart shows the Rocine types, their acid or alkaline food needs, and the percentage of raw foods needed for your health and healing.

- Apply your Type Minerals to the Food Guide

Thin Type Genetics	Acid/Alkaline Genetics	% Food-Ash Needed	%Raw Foods
Atrophic	*Acid*	*80% alkaline*	*90*
Exesthesic	*Acid*	*70% alkaline*	*70*
Marasmic	*Acid*	*60% alkaline*	*50*
Neurogenic	*Acid*	*70% alkaline*	*50*
Pathoferic	*Alkaline*	*50-50*	*30*
Sillevitic	*Alkaline*	*50-50*	*30*

Note: The above percentages vary depending on aging and the health of each individual type.
* You require this Muscle type diet (unless vegetarian).

Muscle Types / Food Guide
Breakfast

[Superimpose the nutritional information from your

EGGS* (1-2) with lettuce, tomato, or salad, whole grain toast; (add bacon or sausage 1-3 times weekly if desired) — 2-4 times/week; or

FRUIT fresh salad, and protein (yogurt, milk, cheeses, seeds, nuts) —1-3 times/week; or

CEREALS, with fruit, seeds, nuts —2-5 times/week; or

OTHER choices — 0-1 times weekly

<u>*Daily liquids:*</u>
Pure water, citrus, vegetable juices, soups, other —as desired
Coffee, teas —0-2 cups

[Include selections from your type mineral needs everyday.]

Muscle Types / Food Guide

<u>*Lunch*</u>

SALADS, *mixed green, protein (poultry, fish, egg, cheese, seeds or nuts, etc.), whole grain breads*
[Dressing: olive oil/vinegar; low-fat, low-cal dressings]
— 2-4 times/week; or

SANDWICH, *whole grains with a protein (cheese, tuna, ham, etc.); and salad and/or vegetables*
— 1-4 times/week; or

POULTRY, FISH, 3-6 oz., with a mixed green salad and/or vegetables
—1-3 times/week; or

OTHER choices (with salad or vegetables)
—1-2 times/week

[Other oils permitted, but less ideal is soybean oil, a common allergen; minimize commercial dressings. Be sure to include two or more selections from your type food lists in your daily food intake. For in-between meal snacks, eat fruit or vegetables with seeds/nuts.]

[Include selections from your type mineral needs everyday.]

Muscle Types / Food Guide
Dinner

POULTRY, FISH *(4-6 oz.), with salad and/or vegetables*
—2-4 times/week; or

PASTA *with protein (chicken, etc.) with salad and/or vegetables*
— 2-4 times/week; or

VEGETARIAN *meal with salad and/or vegetables*
—1-3 times/week; or

LEAN BEEF *(4-6 oz.) with salad and/or vegetables*
— 0-1 times/week

OTHER *choices with salad and/or vegetables*
— 0-1 times/week

Desserts:
Fruits, fresh —as desired
Low-sugar, healthy desserts
— 0-3 times/wk

Food Guide Notes

Steamed Vegetables —

Minerals are lost in the boiling of vegetables; steaming or wok cooking is best.

Food Combinations —

If you have a weak digestive system then eating proteins at the same meal with starches often results in indigestion, gas, or constipation.

Periodic Detox —

You tend to over-indulge in acid-ash foods (proteins and carbohydrates), and often need occasional elimination diets for tissue waste-acid removal. Have a holistic doctor or nutritionist supervise such detox (where you have an alkaline-ash diet along with protein supplementation).

Minimize —

- Fatty foods
- Commercial salad dressings
- Beef, red meats, processed meats
- Coffee, white sugar, corn syrup, alcohol

Vegetarian Proteins —

You require a carnivorous diet. An exception is the *nitropheric* type who functions best with a *vegetarian* diet. The other muscle types are born to be carnivores. It is very difficult for them to be pure vegetarians because of their strong intuitive cravings for fish, poultry, meat, or eggs. If vegetarian, then because of your high needs for amino acids and acid-ash foods, you should take a protein supplement of 25-40 grams/day (powdered protein in juice).

Healthy Weight —

Several of you gain weight as the ravages of age, lack of exercise and dietary excesses take their toll. By eating according to your body type, you should naturally lose excess weight. Each type also has a few individual factors that only apply to them!

You have a good ability to lose weight by following the Food Guide instructions. The most common problem I find with your weight-control is liver and kidney irritation due to food allergies, which results in extra pounds. The key is to eat non-allergic foods.

If drinking more than 3-4 cups daily of coffee or tea, you may have a hypoglycemic problem (low blood sugar), which contributes to making fat, ill-health, and delayed healing. (Refer to the earlier books for help with this healing.)

———

Appendix

Brief Extracts from
"The 22 Unique Body Types"

_____

49

Types
(Brief extract)

Type comes from 'typus' meaning an image or impression, the study of types being called typology.

▶ *Rocine: "A combination of mental and structural features is consistently found in people of the same type."*

Rocine wrote that all types are a mixture of positive and negative qualities. He based his work on the biochemical individuality of our *mineral* absorption and utilization. Of course, all minerals are absorbed, but he postulated that different types of people *selectively* absorb certain minerals, to a greater or lesser extent, requiring specific mineral foods for their enhanced health and healing. This is the basis of his types.

▶ *The type information cannot predict what or who you will become, or how successful or not, but your type is capable of bringing a creative excellence to whatever you do in life. If your type has negative qualities that you disagree with, remember that they are only tendencies and may or may not manifest in you.*

This book enlarges on Rocine's premise (early 1900's), integrated with the later research of Herbert Sheldon, M.D., Ph.D., at Harvard University (1930's), along with my fifty years of observations and experience with this subject.

Comparing your shared physical (and sometimes psychological) descriptions with the Celebrity Lists further assists the identification of your type. It is not that you will look exactly like, or be a twin to, any particular celebrity. Look closely at a celebrity's features: face, profile, height, weight, head, etc. If you know something about their talents, beliefs, success and failure spheres, health and weight challenges, attitudes and behaviors, etc., then you get clues as to what your type may be.

———

Understanding Types and Sub-Types

Each of us has a clearly discernible dominant type. Visualize the celebrity examples from movies, politics, sports, the arts and public life, and try to identify with their physical features. Look for similar features, remembering that you will not recognize all attributes in yourself. You are not looking for your twin!

The sub-type issue is the main reason people of the same major type can look so different. Remember that a type description does not characterize you exactly, but depicts your individual variant of a type.

▶ *The type questionnaire pinpoints the major features of that type: if the celebrity examples are unhelpful, you may be an unusual variant (in which case ignore the celebrity issue and give yourself 7 points on Question 1).*

———

Minerals

Minerals are essential life nutrients that accelerate enzyme and chemical reactions and provide a basis for your body typing. Although found in all tissues, different minerals tend to be concentrated in certain organs, their presence or absence contributing to the healing of such tissues; e.g., zinc accelerates prostate healing; calcium and manganese promote bone, joint and connective tissue healing.

Specific foods nurture each type, some people needing meats for their health others needing a vegetarian diet. A high potassium diet nurtures one person, while another needs high sulfur, calcium, zinc, or another mineral.

Mineral Digestion and Absorption

Compared to vitamins, minerals are *difficult* to digest, absorb, and utilize. In people with strong digestive systems, this aspect may not be important. The following factors should be in place for optimal mineral metabolism:

1. Stomach Hydrochloric Acid Production
2. Parathyroid Hormone Balance
3. Organ Toxic Metal and Chemical Removal
   [See details in <u>The 22 Unique Body Types.</u>]

———

Total Body Healing

Note that from a holistic healing perspective, in addition to minerals and type information, observe these healing factors:

> *Nutrient Balance*
> *Mental Balance*
> *Emotional Balance*
> *Spiritual Balance*
> *Detoxifying Integrity*

The above factors are all important to your total healing especially if you are interested in self-healing (see my earlier books).

———

Appendix B

Researchers
(Brief extract)

The predominant workers in this area of human individuality from around 1880's to the 1960's are Herbert Sheldon, M.D., Ph.D., Roger Williams, Ph.D., and Victor Rocine, D.Sc.

Much information on Sheldon's research exists on-line and in medical psychology libraries; for interested readers there are other lines of research published in the last century. This present book is primarily about Rocine's body types.

Herbert Sheldon M.D., Ph.D.

In contrast to Rocine, Sheldon at Harvard University in the 1930's was trained in the scientific method and did painstaking research and publishing on human individuality. In comparing his findings with Rocine's work, a direct putative correlation is visible.

Roger J. Williams, Ph.D.

Another significant researcher in human individuality is the renowned scientist and biochemist, Roger J. Williams. He demonstrated that different people have varying levels of nutrients, enzymes, and other metabolic chemicals in their bloodstreams.

▶ *Williams's research firmly expands on the premise of individual nutritional needs in human beings. If interested in his research, I highly recommend his book <u>Biochemial Individuality</u>.*

Victor Rocine, D.Sc.

Note that when a negative feature is indicated, say neurotic tendencies, all members of the type are <u>not</u> that way; it is a type tendency reported by Rocine.

Rocine studied type-related diseases finding links between mineral and dietary factors with individual types and their diseases. In each body type, one or more dominant minerals are preferentially absorbed and utilized over other minerals.

He recognized discrete body types from their physical appearance finding genetically based mineral dominance to be the determining feature. He also correlated their physical features with psychological characteristics.

Appendix C

Genetics, Types, and Diet
(Brief extract)

This section deals with how nervous system genetics helps determine your eating choices for health: you are either born to be a predominant meat eater, a partial or complete vegetarian, or something between the two. The genetic factor determining this dietary aspect is the *sympathetic and parasympathetic* components of your central nervous system. This represents a basic factor in eating for health.

This chapter helps you understand your dietary inheritance, although instinctively, you may already have arrived there!

- If born **sympathetic** dominant you are *genetically acid*, desiring a predominantly *vegetarian* diet for your health (about 70% fruit, salad, vegetables to 30% proteins and carbohydrates).

- If born **parasympathetic** dominant you are *genetically alkaline*, desiring a predominantly *carnivorous* diet for your health (70% proteins, carbohydrates). Few of you ever choose to become vegetarian because of the difficulty in satisfying your protein needs.

- If born ***intermediate*** dominant you may eat food groups with little concern for the acid/alkaline factor. However, after age 40, you need a semi-vegetarian diet for healthy eating.

———

Chart of Relative Nervous System Dominance

In the following Chart, if you relate to many of the symptoms on one side you probably have that nervous system dominance; relating to both sides indicates *Intermediate* dominance.

If Vegetarian (Over-acid)
Eat 70% fruits, salads, vegetables
And 30% proteins, carbohydrates

If Carnivore (Over-alkaline)
Eat 70% proteins, carbohydrates
And 30% fruits, salads, vegetables

If Intermediate
Eat 50:50 of acid and alkaline-ash foods

Make an *approximate* estimate of your daily acid and alkaline food intake (such ratios varying from type to type).

———

Symptoms of Relative Genetic Dominance

Vegetarians (Over-acid)	*Carnivores* (Over-alkaline)
Sympathetic Dominance	*Parasympathetic Dominance*
little or no flesh desire	desire flesh
easily constipated	rarely constipated
slow digestion	fast digestion
easily dehydrated	not dehydrated
strong thirst	low thirst
pale face	flushed face
high pulse after food	slow pulse after food
easy gag reflex	slow gag reflex
cool dry skin	moist warm skin
nervous stomach	calm stomach
little eyelid blinking	much blinking
nervous tendency	mostly calm
slower healing	faster healing
low oxygen-uptake	good oxygen-uptake
easily breathless	seldom breathless
insomnia common	sleep easier
few muscle cramps	some night cramps
calcium deposits rare	get calcium deposits

Help Identifying your Body Type with Dr. Stenbeck

If you desire help in identifying your body type, follow these instructions, and answer the questionnaire. For further information and fees, send me an email from page one of the website:

DrStenbeck.net

First name: _____

Country of birth: _____

Upload photos and send to the above website:

- Head and shoulders: front and side views

- Full body: front and side views

- Also 1-2 teenage views

- If possible, casual photos of mother, father, siblings

MY TYPE CLASS MAY BE: _____

   (Thin, Muscle, or Fat)

AGE   -   _____

HEIGHT   -   _____ feet/inches

MY WEIGHT - _____ pounds

    - Heaviest at age: _____

    - Lightest as adult: _____

    - Estimate age 15: _____

VISION - Excellent   Average   Poor:

HAIR -   Natural color: _____

    - Thin/thick? _____

    - balding? _____

SKIN - Quality: _____

    - History of acne, boils, other:

_____

TEETH -   Strong   Weak   Dentures

 - Cavity history: Many   Moderate Few

MUSCLES -   Strong   Average   Weak

      Sports played _____

JOINTS -   Strong   Average   Weak

HEALTH - Childhood diseases?

_____

_____

    - Adult diseases?

_____

AVERAGE DIET

- Beef _____ (times/week)

- Poultry _____ (times/week)

- Fish _____ (times/week)

- Eggs _____ (times/week)

- Water _____ (glasses/day):

- Vegetarian? Vegan? _____

- Other? _____

- Did your childhood diet differ? _____

The above will help me know who you are! I will send you a follow-up questionnaire for further help in identifying your body type.

Appendix E

On-line Health Consultation with Dr. Stenbeck

For further information, or to comment on this book, or to receive a response on any health issue from a holistic viewpoint, send an email inquiry from page one of my website:

DrStenbeck.net

Following that, I will suggest further healing needs, which we may pursue with an on-line consult.

———

Appendix F

Notes

See *The 22 Unique Body Types,* available at the usual online source, for further information and details on all of the 22 Types. The Appendix in that book also has more information about:

- *Mineral Functions and Food Sources*

- *Further Reading*